In My World

A Winter Wonderland

LAURA BOWLEY

Copyrighted Material
In My World: A Winter Wonderland
Copyright © 2025 Laura Bowley. All Rights Reserved.
Published by Synergy Communications
No part of this publication may be reproduced, stored in a retrieval system or transmitted, in any form or by any means – electronic, mechanical, photocopying, recording or otherwise – without prior written permission from the publisher, except for the inclusion of brief quotations in a review.

For information about this title or to order other books and/or electronic media,
contact the publisher:
Laura Bowley
brightreads.ca
laura@brightreads.ca

ISBNs:
print: 978-0-9949447-3-3
eBook: 978-0-9949447-2-6
Printed in the United States of America

With thanks to 1106 Design (1106design.com) for their original cover and page design concepts for the *In My World* series of books.

Download the discussion guide for this book at brightreads.ca.

Photo Credits
Cover: *Red Benches in the fog in winter* | By Jaroslaw Grudzinski | Adobe Stock
    Story 1: Carmen Keuper | Unsplash
    Story 2: AI Generated
    Story 3: Judi Jutras | Pexels
    Story 4: Yan Krukov | Pexels
    Story 5: Ethan Hu | Unsplash
    Story 6: Filip Mroz | Unsplash
    Story 7: Keith Jonson | Unsplash
    Story 8: Dmytro | Adobe Stock
    Story 9: Jenko Ataman | Adobe Stock
    Story 10: S Wloczyk | Pixabay
    Story 11: Will Tu | Adobe Stock
    Story 12: Asad Photo | Pexels

A Winter Wonderland

Story 1: The Snowflake

Story 2: A Day on the Slopes

Story 3: A Snowy Path

Story 4: Winter Adventures

Story 5: The Snowman

Story 6: Winter Chores

Story 7: Snow Angels

Story 8: A Skating Party

Story 9: Making Cookies

Story 10: A Warm Fire

Story 11: Dive In!

Story 12: A Winter Getaway

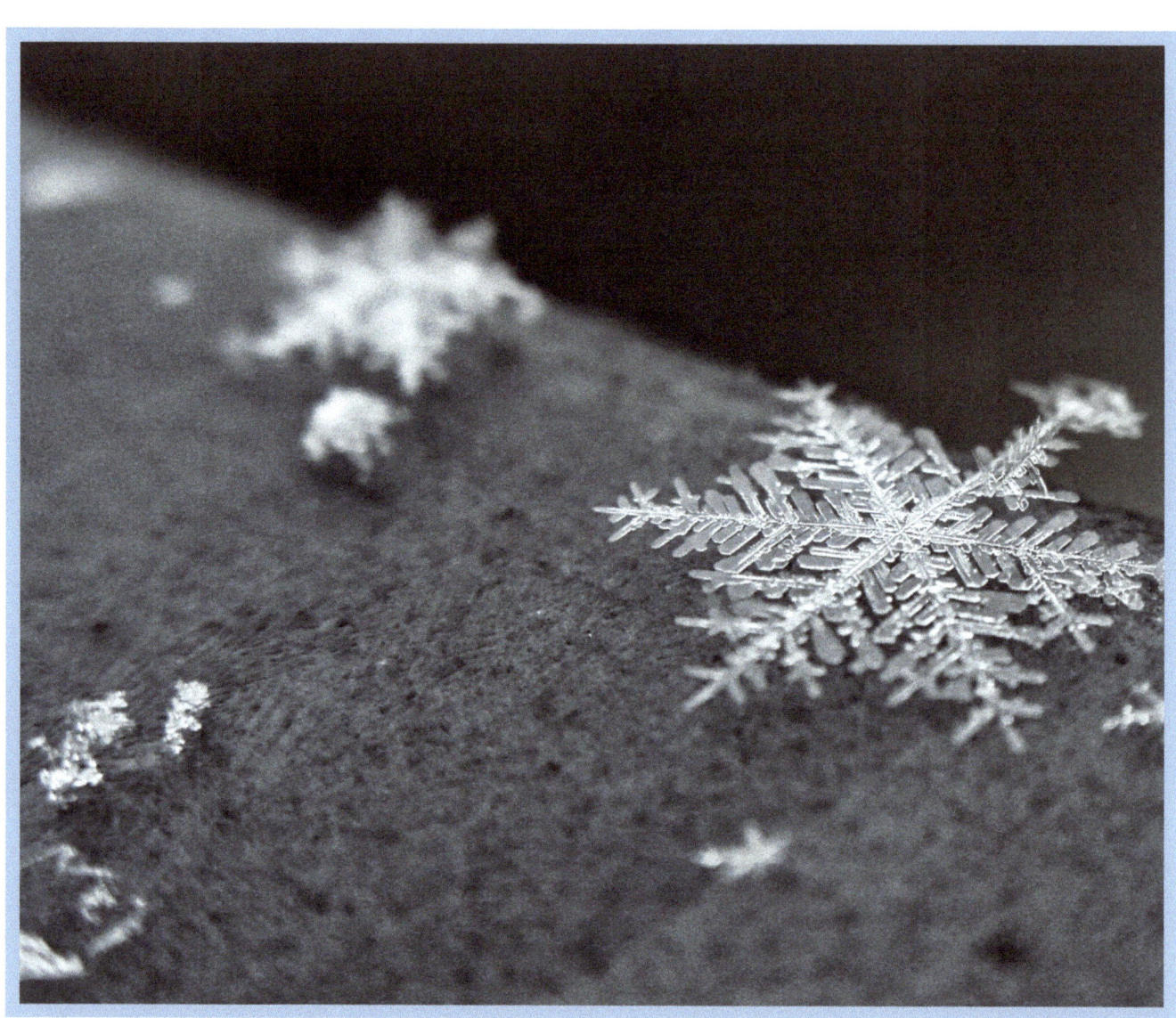

The Snowflake

The snowflake is a tiny masterpiece of nature. Each delicate branch is perfectly formed. No two are alike, making every snowflake a marvel. It rests softly on a cool surface, waiting to melt or drift away.

Have you ever caught a snowflake on your glove?

Have you ever stopped to admire its beauty?

Snowflakes remind us of the quiet magic in winter's cold embrace. What do you find magical about snow?

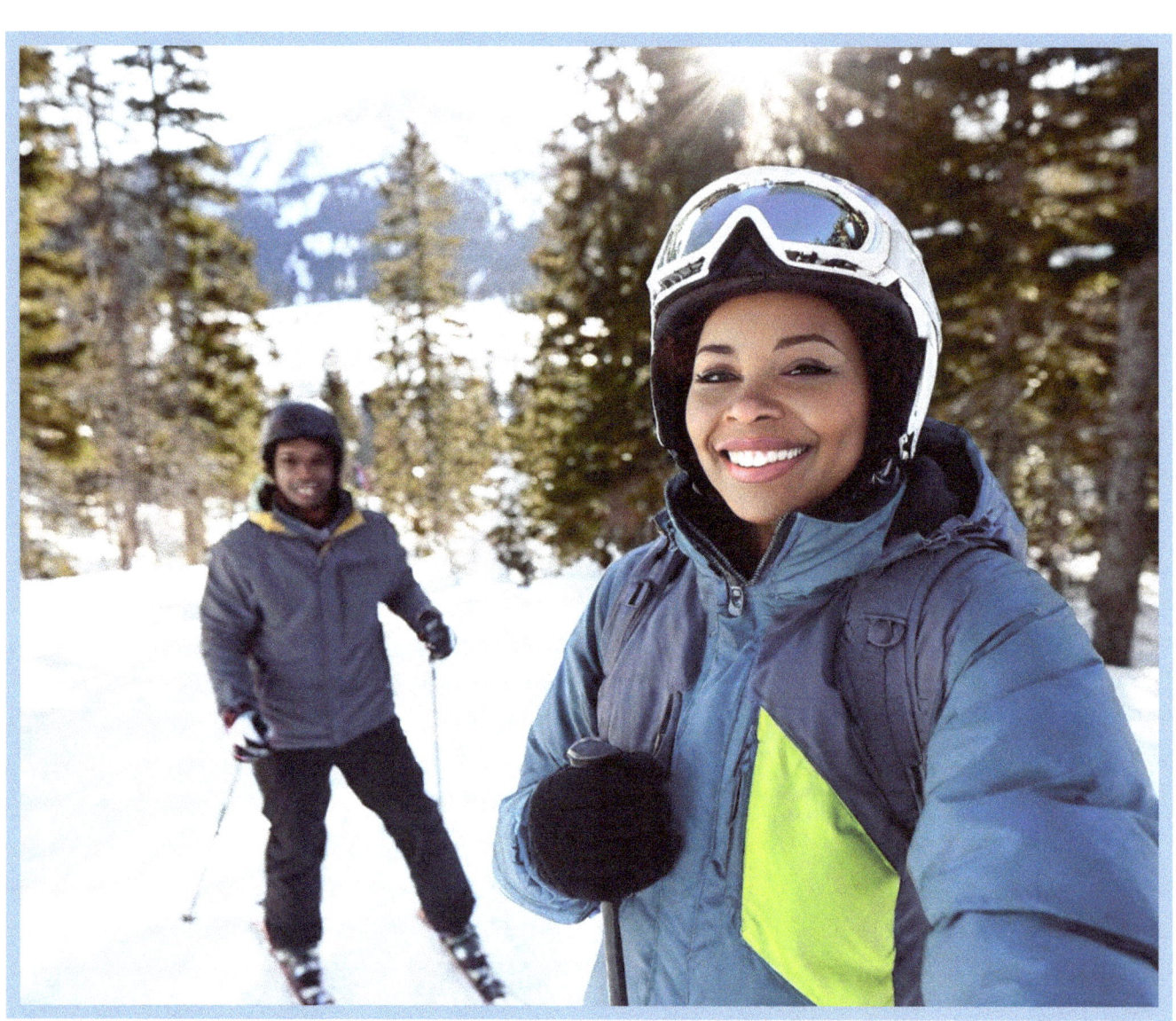

STORY 2

A Day on the Slopes

The air feels crisp and fresh on a sunny winter day. These skiers are having so much fun, gliding down the snowy hill with big smiles. The sunlight sparkles on the snow, and the swoosh of skis mixes with laughter. Can you imagine the cold breeze on your face?

After skiing, they head to the cozy ski lodge to warm up by a crackling fire. Maybe they'll sip hot chocolate with marshmallows or share stories about their favourite runs. Winter days like this are perfect for adventure and relaxing with friends.

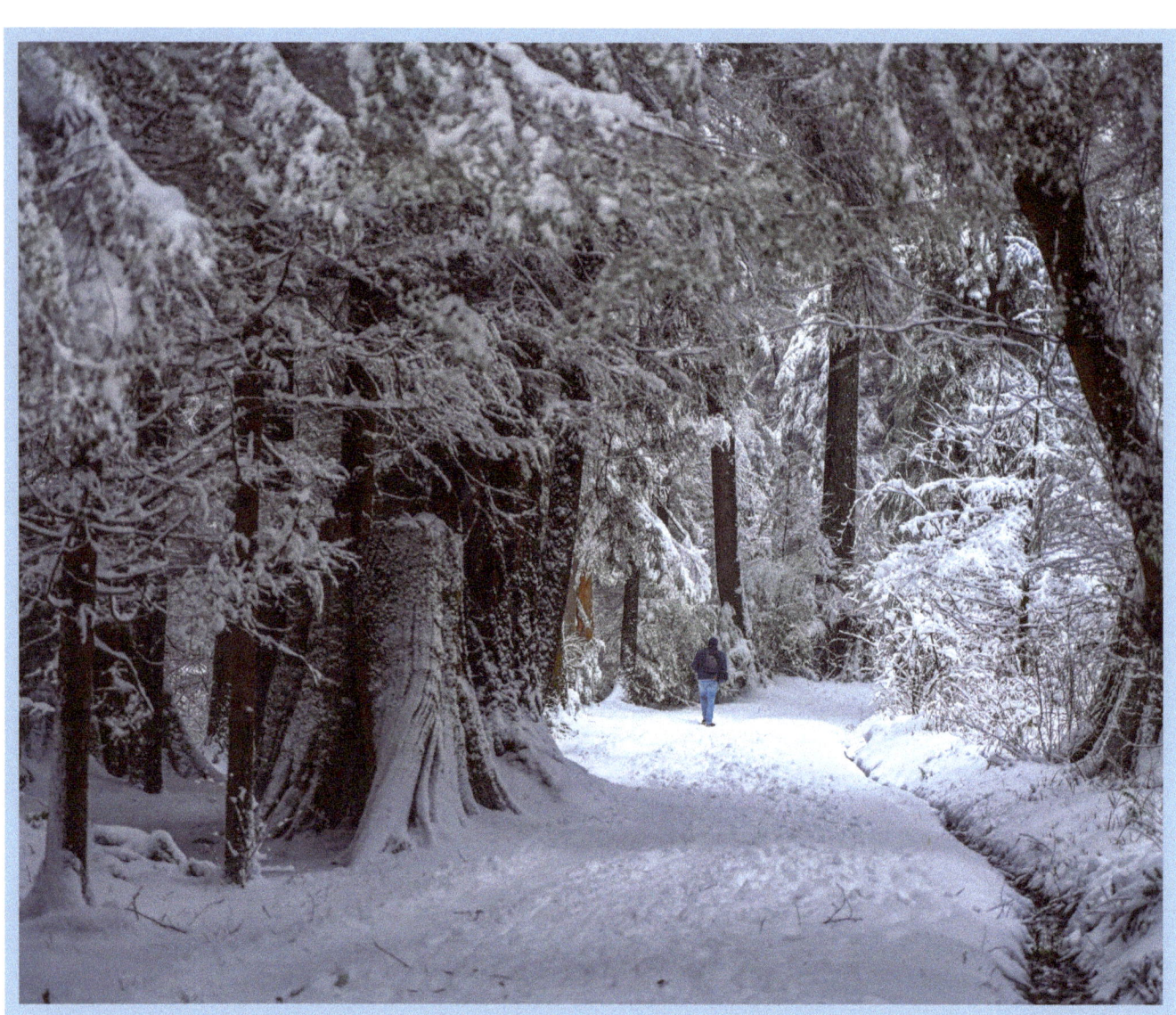

A Snowy Path

The world looks so peaceful after a fresh snowfall.

Trees stand tall, their branches wrapped in white. The path stretches ahead, covered in soft snow. Can you hear the crunch of snow underfoot? The air is crisp and smells of pine.

The forest feels magical in the stillness. Deer may have left tiny hoofprints in the snow. A bird might perch high above, blending with the branches. Winter slows everything down. It invites us to pause and admire its quiet beauty.

Walking this snowy path feels special. The world seems to hold its breath. It's as if winter is waiting to share its secrets with us.

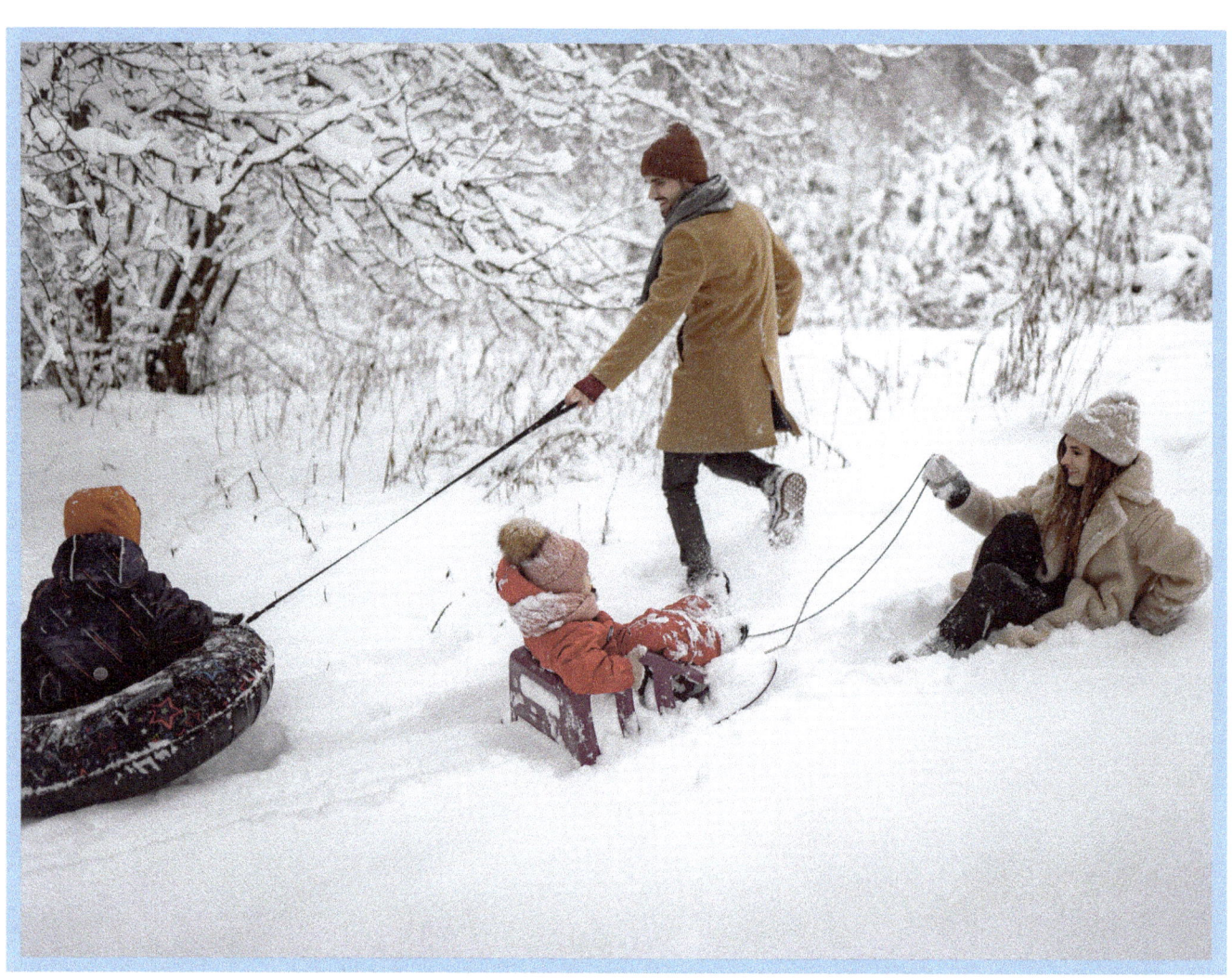

STORY 4

Winter Adventures

The fresh snow is perfect for a winter adventure! A family enjoys a day together in the woods. The kids are bundled up in warm coats, hats, and scarves. Their laughter fills the cold air.

The father pulls his child on a snow tube through the soft, white powder. The mother sits in the snow, smiling as she holds the rope of the sled. Her cozy fur-lined coat and knitted hat keep her warm as she watches her family have fun. The snow-covered trees and quiet forest make everything feel magical, like they're in a winter wonderland.

Snowflakes fall softly, adding to the beauty of the day. Everyone's cheeks are rosy from the cold. They are making happy memories and enjoying a snowy day together.

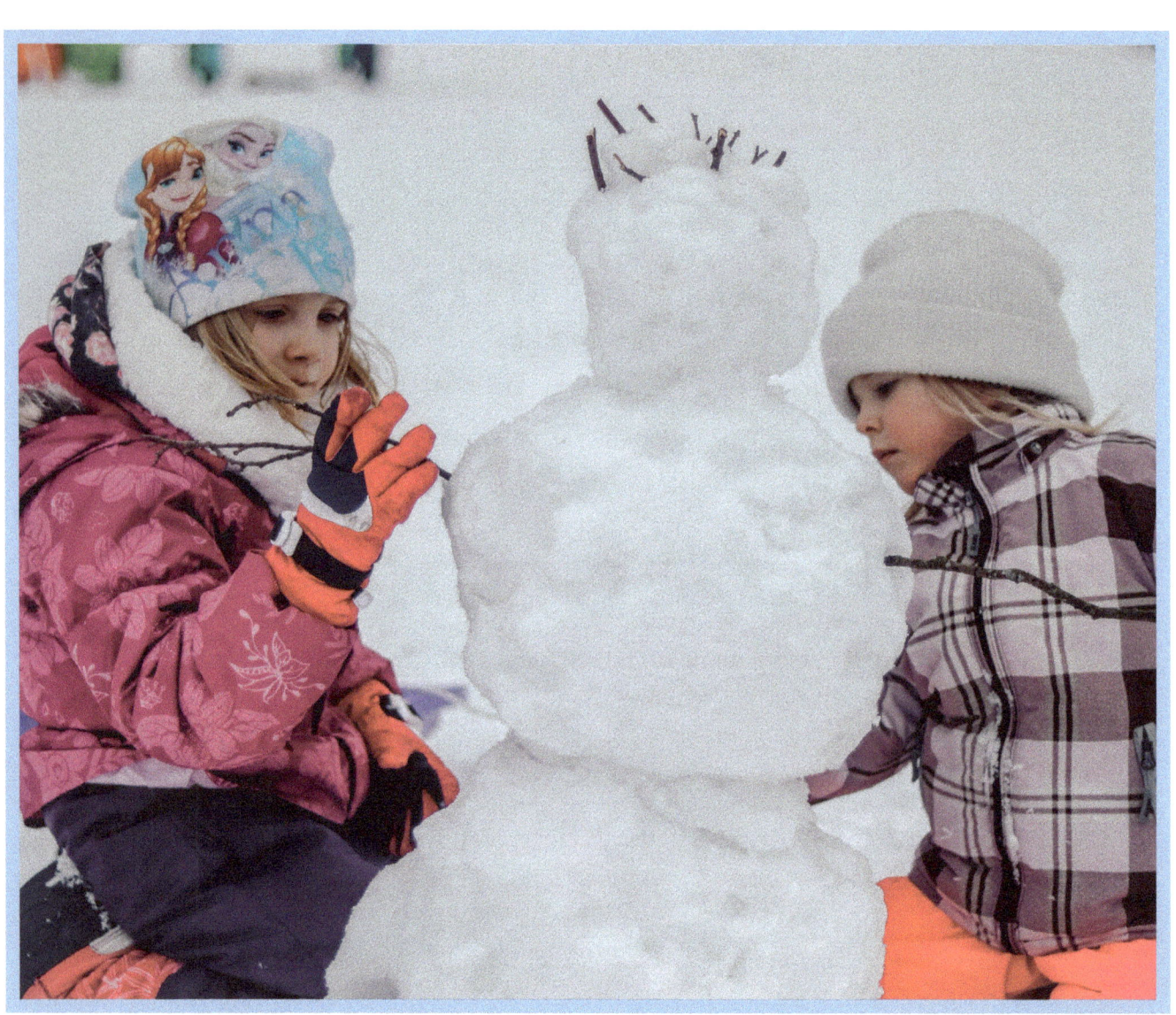

STORY 5

The Snowman

Building a snowman is one of the best parts of winter! Two girls work together, carefully shaping the snow into three big balls. One girl places twigs for arms and sticks in the top for spiky hair. The other girl makes sure everything looks just right. Their gloves and warm coats keep them cozy as they build their frosty friend.

The snowman's round face is almost done, ready for a big smile and maybe even a carrot nose. The girls laugh and chat while they work, leaving little footprints in the snow. The snowy day feels full of fun.

When their snowman is finished, it will stand proudly in the snow, like a winter sculpture made by two best friends. Building a snowman is more than just a fun activity—it's a way to make lasting memories on a chilly day!

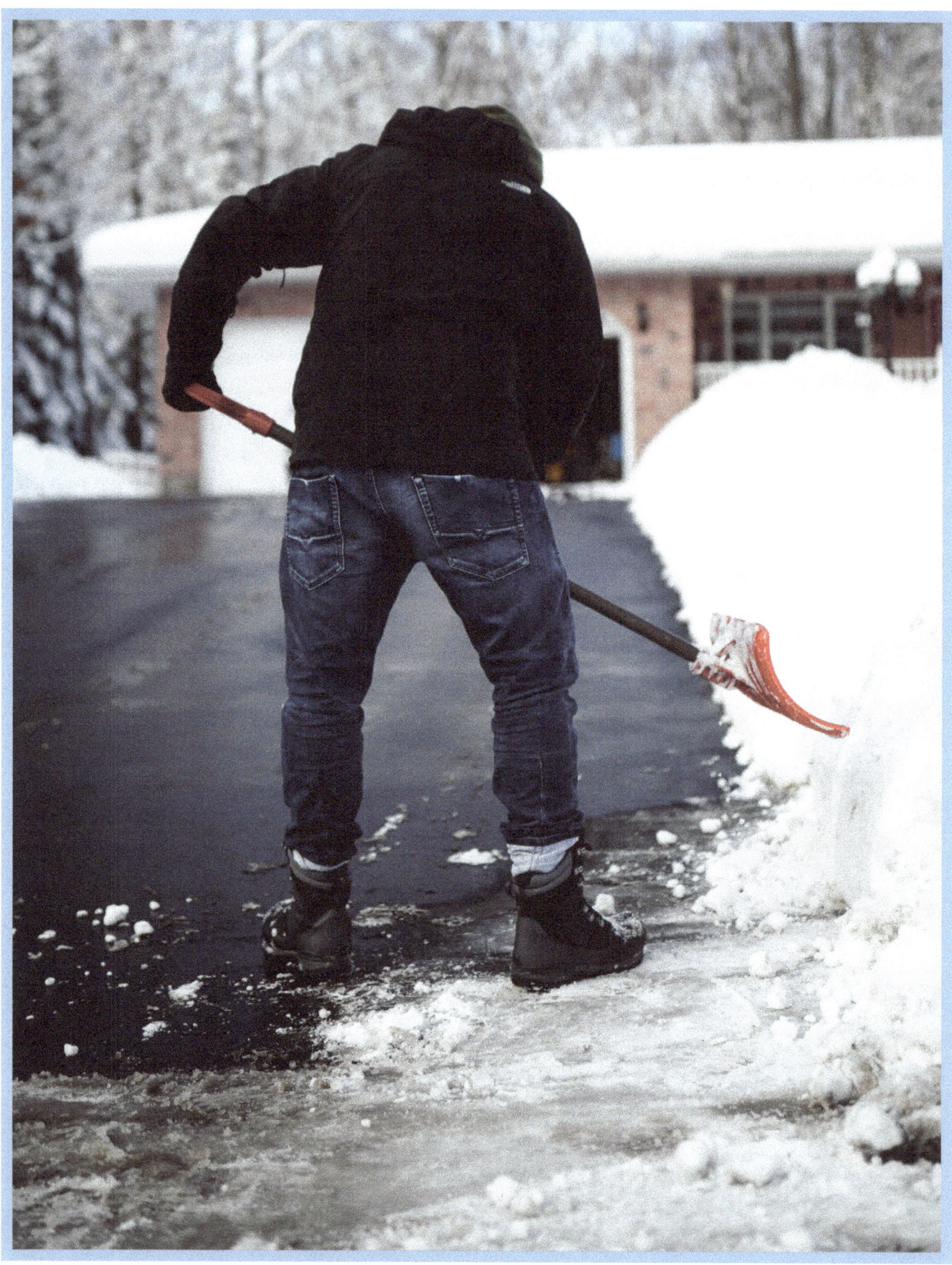

STORY 6

Winter Chores

Shoveling snow is more than just work—it's part of what makes winter special. With each scoop, you clear a path through the fresh, white snow, keeping your home safe and ready for visitors. The sound of the shovel and the cold air on your face remind you of the beauty of winter all around.

It's a good time to stop and look at the snowy trees and feel proud of the job you're doing. Even though it's hard work, it feels good to finish and see the clean driveway, knowing you've made a difference. And shovelling snow is good exercise!

Shoveling isn't just about clearing snow—it's about taking care of the people and places that matter most. It's one of those small tasks that feels meaningful when you stand back and see the clear path you've created, ready for the next steps forward.

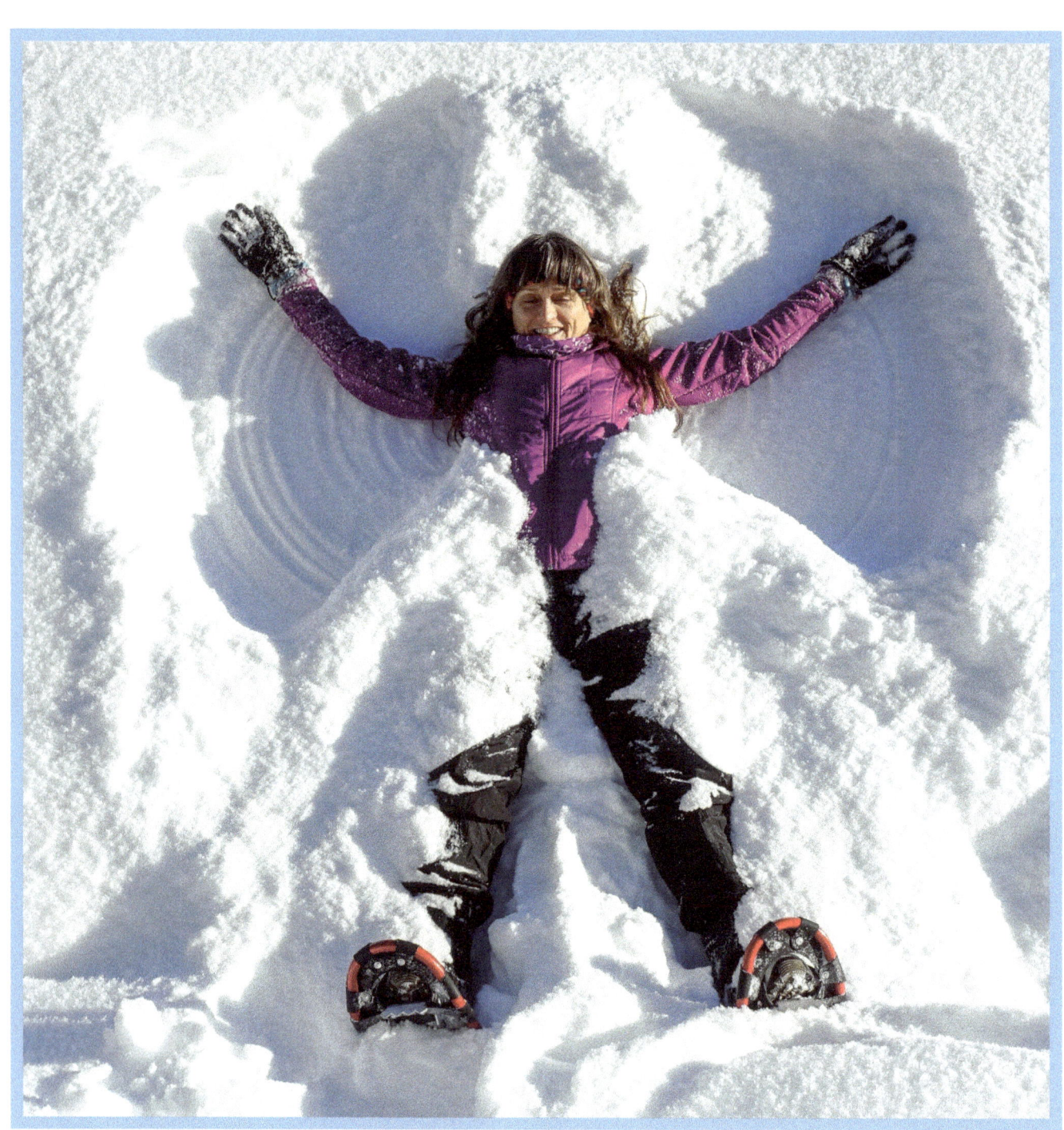

Snow Angels

Have you ever made a snow angel?

An expanse of bright, white snow, where no one has walked before, is an invitation to make a snow angel. Turn around and flop down in the snow! As you sink into the snow, you feel the cold on your back.

Wave your arms up and down to make the wings. Move your legs from side to side to make the angel's skirt. Moving your legs is hard when the snow is deep!

Before you stand up to admire your handiwork, take a moment to enjoy the cold, crisp air and the warmth of the sun on your face. Gaze up at the fluffy snow on the trees. Hear the silence of a snowy day.

Now, carefully step out of your snowy masterpiece and admire the angel you've created!

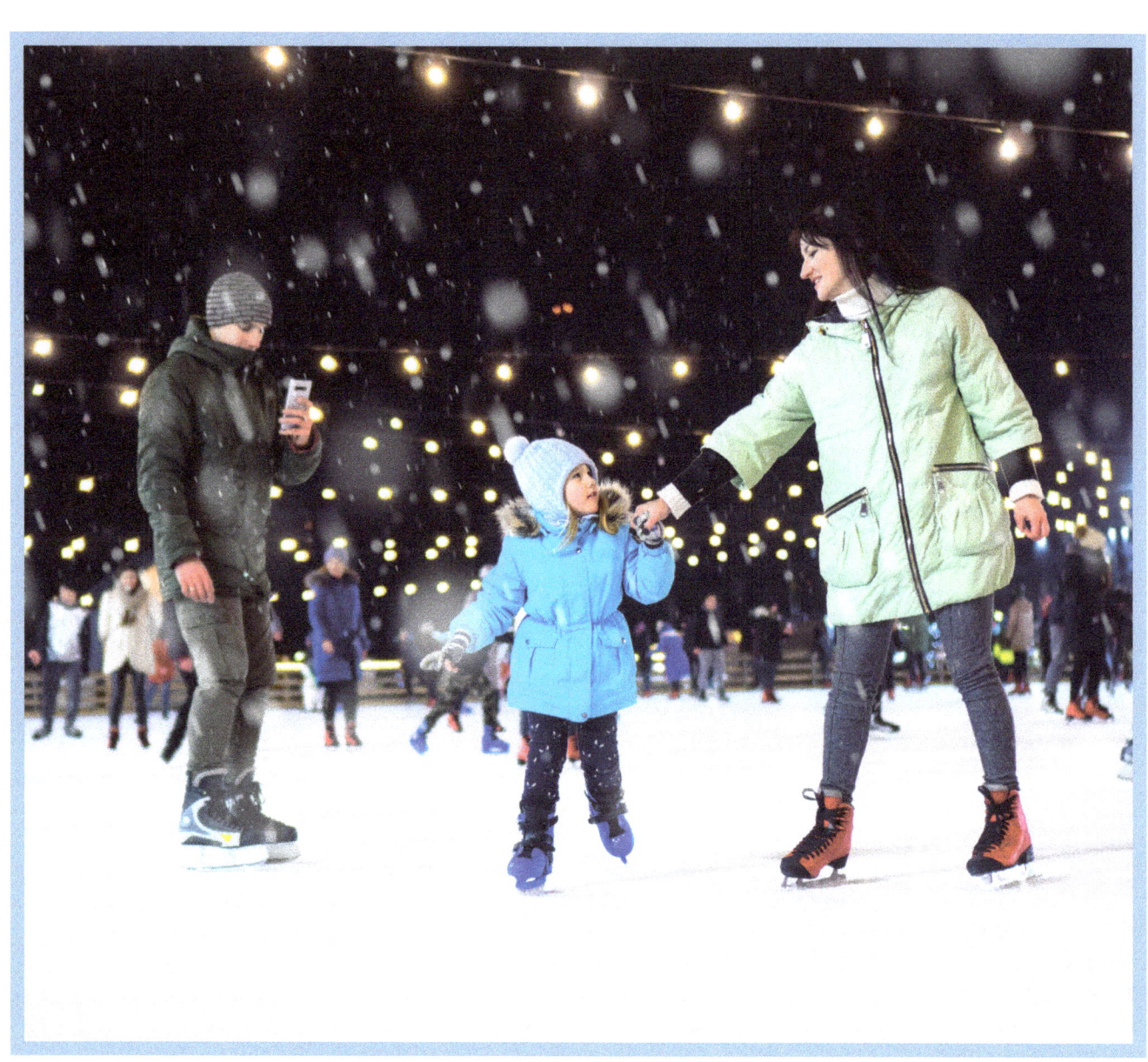

STORY 8

A Skating Party

Time to celebrate! The rink is frozen and the ice is clear of snow. After putting their skates on, the skaters stand up carefully and take a few steps. Yay, they didn't fall down! Soon, they get the hang of it, gliding around the ice, arms swinging to propel them forward.

One girl holds her mother's hand, just in case she slips and falls. It's her first time on skates! Her proud father takes photos to remember this special time.

Can you hear the sound of the skate blades on ice? Feel the cold, crisp air on your face? After skating, there's a bonfire to warm up before heading home. Someone has brought hot apple cider to share and marshmallows, chocolate, and graham crackers to make Smores. Let's find a stick and roast some marshmallows!

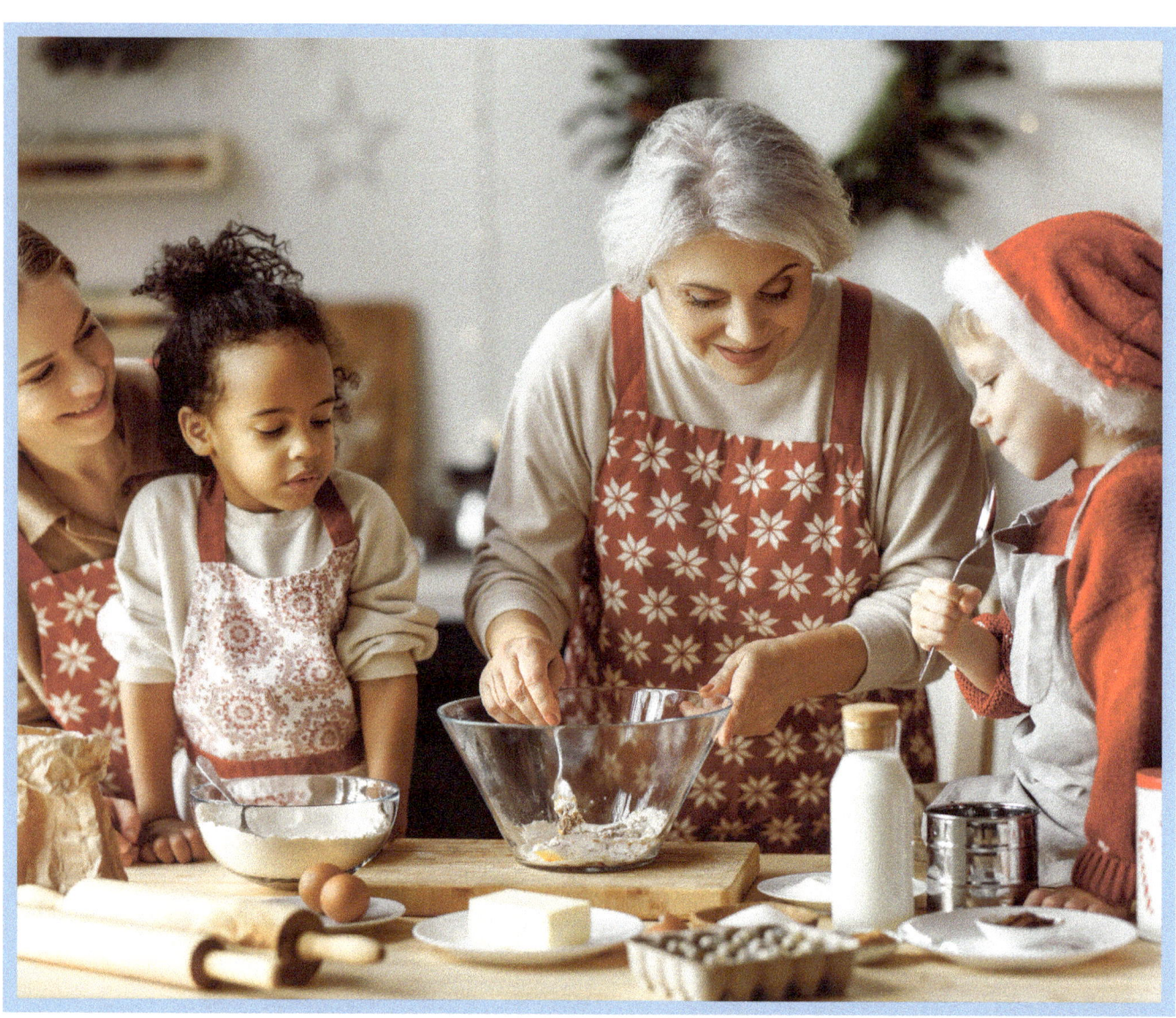

Making Cookies

A family gathers in a cozy kitchen, baking together during the holiday season. Everyone is wearing festive aprons, and the counters are filled with baking ingredients like flour, eggs, and butter. The little boy, dressed as Santa, looks excited as he holds a spoon, ready to help. Are they making cookies, a pie, or tarts?

The young girl, standing next to her mom, looks eager to join in. The mom and grandma share warm smiles, making the scene feel joyful and full of love. Holiday decorations add a festive touch.

Whether they're baking cookies or a cake, the family is making memories that will last a lifetime. The warm light and happy faces show how special these small moments can be.

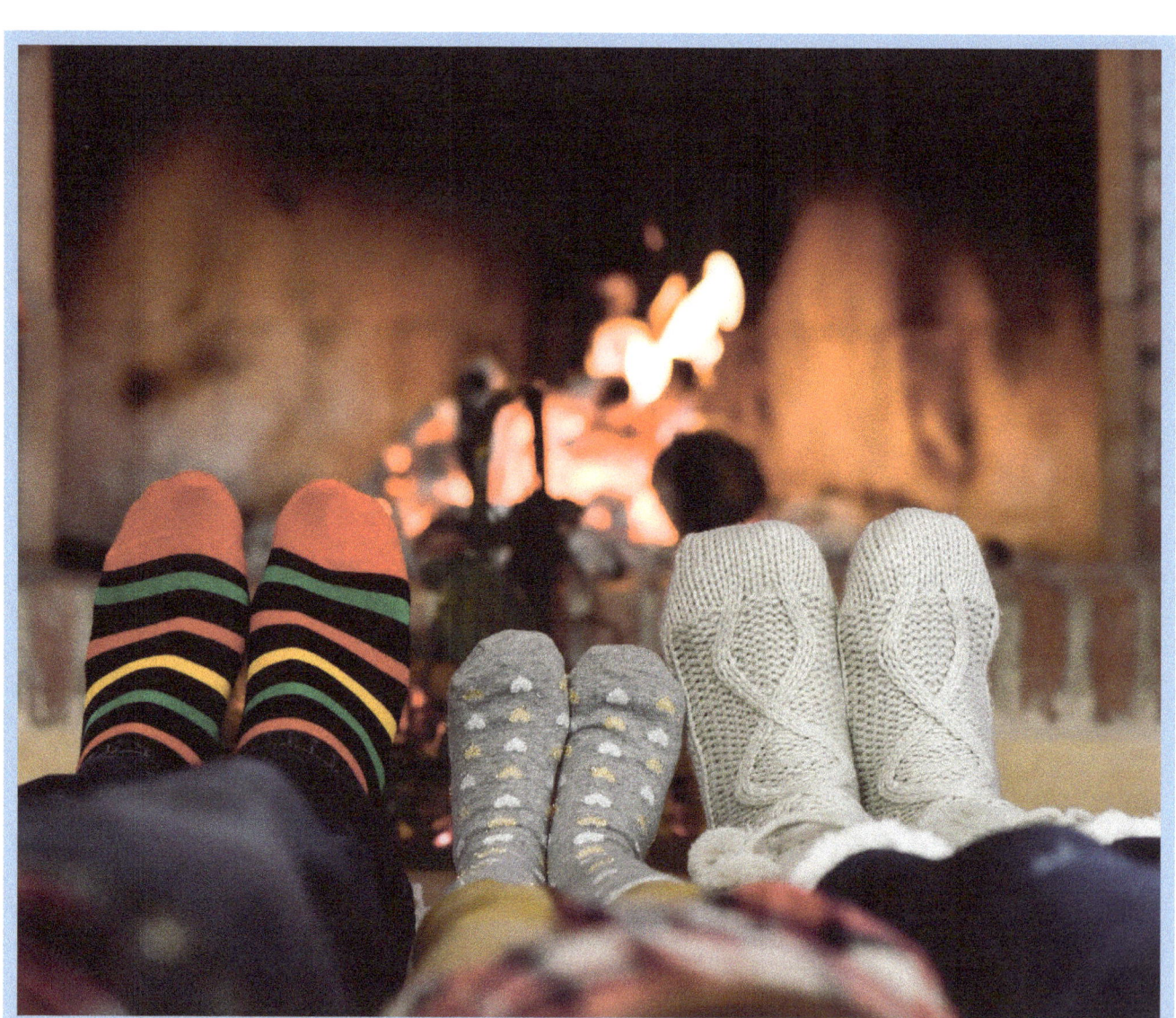

STORY 10

A Warm Fire

Cozying up by the fire is the perfect way to spend a chilly winter evening. Three pairs of feet rest in front of a warm, glowing fireplace. Each pair wears fun, comfy socks—one has colourful stripes, one has tiny hearts, and one is bundled in thick, knit slippers. The crackling flames make the room feel snug and peaceful.

Surrounded by the soft glow of the fire, it's a moment for relaxing and being together. Maybe they're sipping hot cocoa, telling stories, or just enjoying the quiet warmth. The soft flicker of light on the brick fireplace adds a festive touch to the scene.

It's these small, special moments—sharing laughter, warmth, and time with loved ones—that make winter nights so magical.

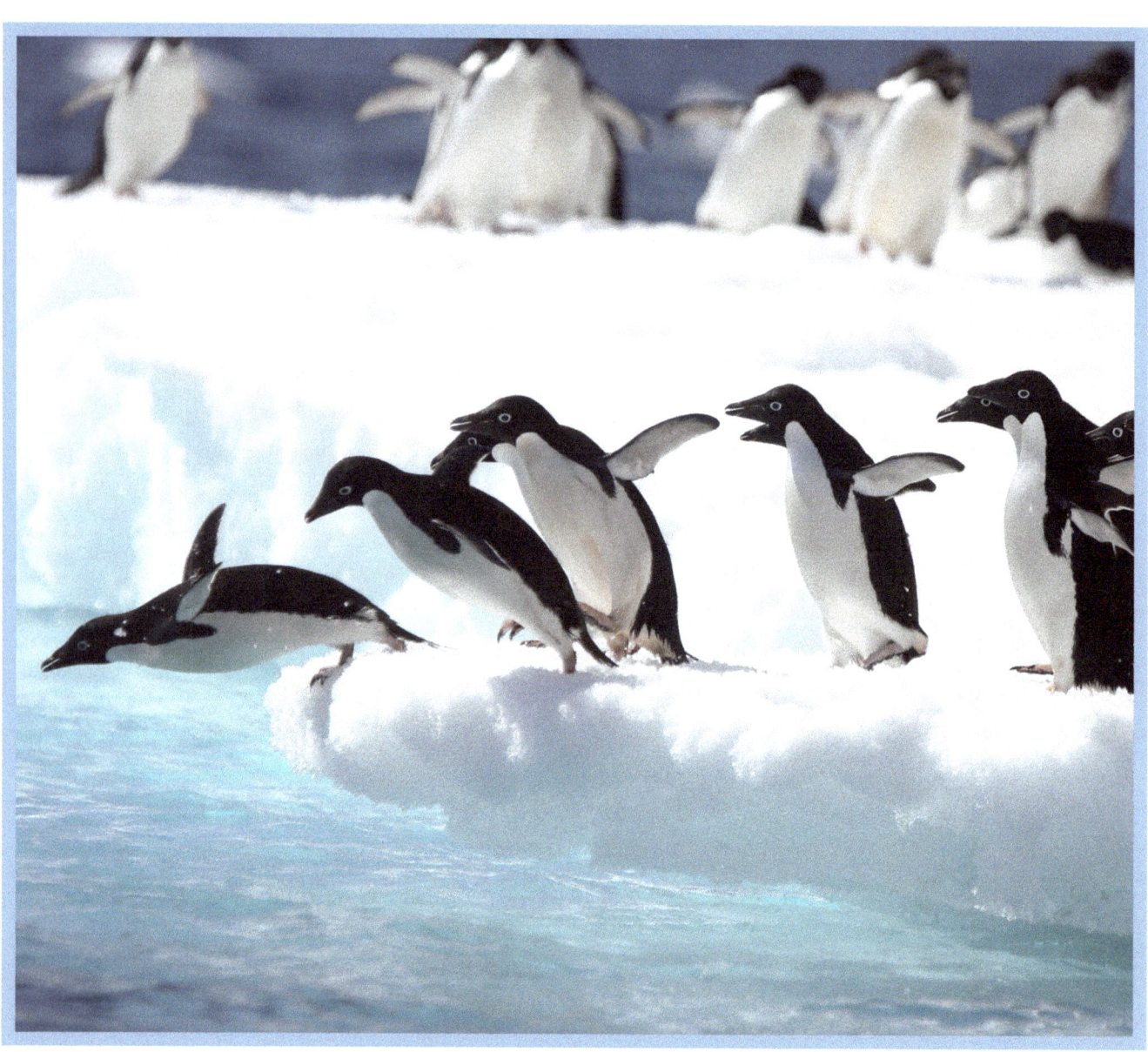

STORY 11

Dive In!

On a bright, icy day, a group of penguins stands together on a snowy edge, ready to take a dive into the cold, blue water below. The first brave penguin has already leapt, while others wait their turn, flapping their wings for balance. Their black-and-white feathers shine against the white snow and the sparkling ocean.

In the background, more penguins waddle around, watching or waiting for their chance to jump. They look excited, as if they're playing or exploring together. The icy scene feels full of energy and teamwork as these adorable birds enjoy their chilly home.

This picture shows how penguins stick together, even in their icy world. Whether they're diving, swimming, or standing in line, they seem to have fun doing it as a group!

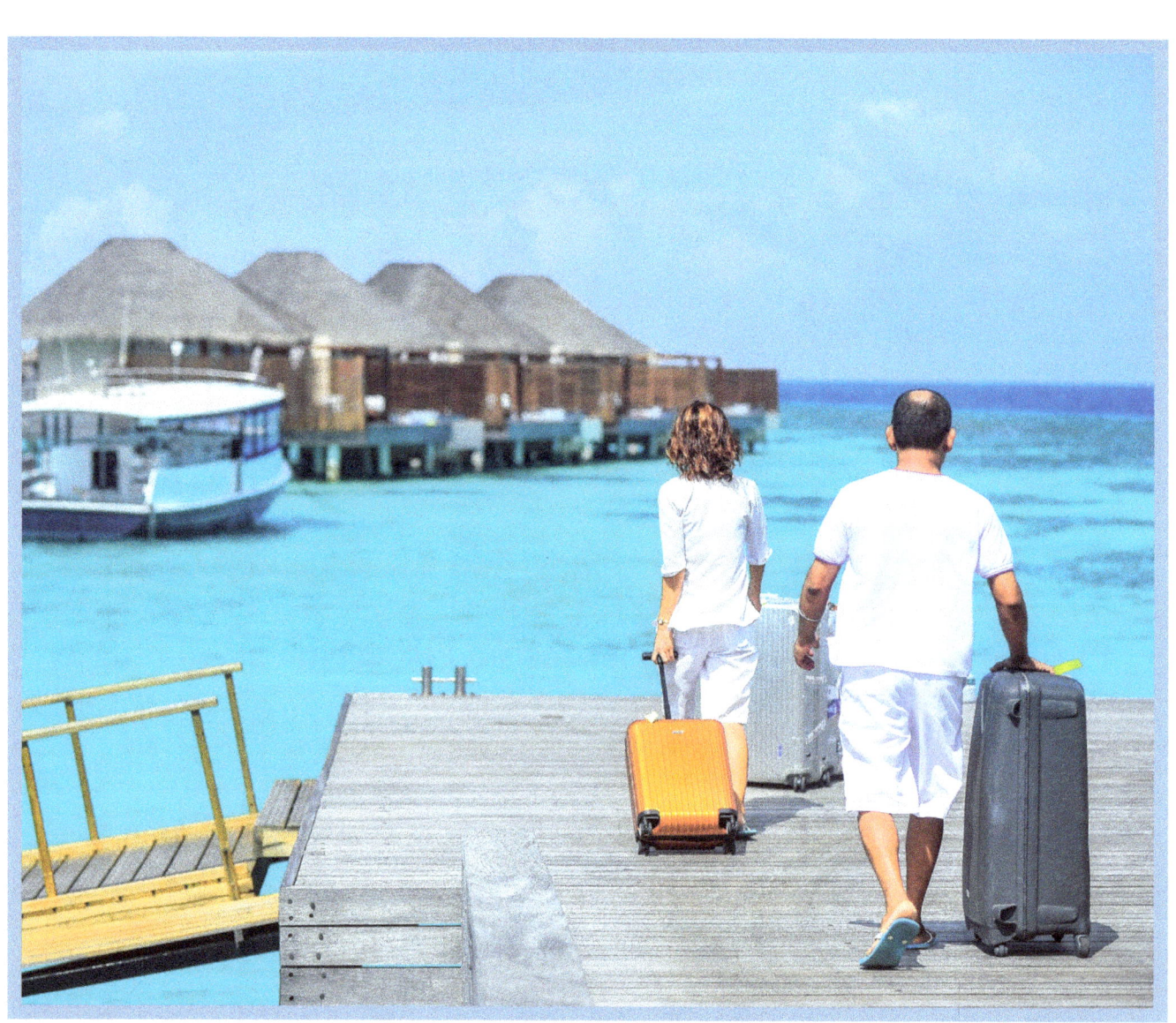

A Winter Getaway

The sun shines bright and warm. The turquoise water sparkles like a dream. A couple walks along the dock with suitcases in hand. Can you feel their excitement?

A winter vacation is a chance to leave the cold and the rush of life behind. It's time to slow down. Soak in the sun. Let the gentle waves wash your cares away. Imagine stepping into your overwater bungalow, the ocean stretching endlessly before you.

What would you do first? Jump into the clear water? Sip a cold drink under the palms? Or sit back and enjoy the view? Whatever you do, let the sun and adventure fill your heart.

www.ingramcontent.com/pod-product-compliance
Lightning Source LLC
Chambersburg PA
CBHW040226040426
42333CB00054B/3454